Pomegranate Tree Guide for Beginners

How to Maintain a Pomegranate Tree

By

Moray Caelan

Table of Contents

CHAPTER 1

Introduction

1.1 What are Pomegranate Trees?

Pomegranate trees, scientifically known as Punica granatum, are deciduous shrubs or small trees that belong to the family Lythraceae. Renowned for their vibrant, ruby-red fruits and ornamental value, these trees have a rich historical and cultural significance dating back centuries.

Botanical Characteristics:

Pomegranate trees typically grow between 15 to 30 feet in height, although some dwarf varieties exist for smaller spaces. They have glossy, narrow leaves that are about 3 to 7 centimeters long and bear striking, trumpet-shaped scarlet flowers, often contrasting beautifully against the dark green foliage.

Fruit Formation and Appearance:

The hallmark of the pomegranate tree is its fruit—a spherical to slightly hexagonal fruit with a tough, leathery outer rind, which encases numerous juicy arils. These arils, containing the seeds and sweet-tart juice, are the edible part of the fruit and range in color from deep red to pink or even white depending on the variety. The interior of the fruit is divided by membranous walls, creating compartments filled with these jewel-like arils.

Cultural Significance:

Pomegranates hold significant cultural and symbolic meanings across various civilizations. They've been revered in ancient mythology, literature, and religious texts for their association with fertility, abundance, and eternal life. For instance, in Greek mythology, the pomegranate symbolizes regeneration and prosperity, while in some cultures, it's a token of good luck or fertility.

Historical Importance:

The history of the pomegranate tree is extensive, tracing back to regions around modern-day Iran and Northern India. Its cultivation spread throughout the Mediterranean, Middle East, and parts of Asia, becoming a staple in various cuisines and medicinal practices. In many cultures, the fruit and its tree have been revered for their medicinal properties, being used to treat ailments ranging from digestive issues to skin problems.

Culinary and Medicinal Uses:

Beyond their cultural and symbolic significance, pomegranates are celebrated for their culinary versatility and health benefits. The arils are used in a variety of dishes, from salads and desserts to beverages, lending their unique sweet-tart flavor and vibrant color. Moreover, pomegranates are a rich source of antioxidants, vitamins, and other nutrients, contributing to their status as a "superfood."

Modern Cultivation:

Today, pomegranate trees are cultivated in diverse regions around the world, with variations in climate impacting the types of cultivars grown. Commercially, their popularity continues to grow due to increased interest in healthy eating and natural remedies. Modern agricultural practices, including hybridization and improved cultivation techniques, have led to the development of new varieties optimized for specific climates and purposes.

Pomegranate trees stand not only as a bearer of delicious and nutritious fruits but also as a symbol of cultural heritage, historical significance, and natural beauty. Their enduring presence in mythology, their widespread cultivation, and their multitude of uses ensure that these trees remain cherished and respected in various facets of human life.

1.2 History and Cultural Significance

The history and cultural significance of pomegranates are as rich as the fruit itself, spanning centuries and weaving through various civilizations, myths, rituals, and traditions.

Ancient Roots:

The origins of pomegranates trace back to regions in modern-day Iran and Northern India, where they were cultivated thousands of years ago. Their cultivation and prominence spread through trade routes across the Mediterranean, Middle East, and Asia, leading to their integration into the cultures of ancient civilizations like Persia, Egypt, Greece, and Rome.

Symbolism and Mythology:

Pomegranates have held symbolic value in many mythologies. In Greek mythology, the story of Persephone eating pomegranate seeds ties her to the underworld, leading to the cycle of seasons. The fruit symbolizes fertility, life, and rebirth in various cultures. Its abundant seeds are often seen as a representation of prosperity and unity.

Religious Significance:

The pomegranate has appeared in religious texts and traditions across different faiths. In Judaism, it's believed that the fruit contains 613 seeds, representing the 613 commandments in the Torah. In Christianity, it symbolizes resurrection and eternal life. In Islamic tradition, it's mentioned in the Quran as a symbol of righteousness.

Art, Literature, and Culture:

Pomegranates have permeated art, literature, and cultural practices worldwide. They've been depicted in paintings, sculptures, and textiles, symbolizing fertility, abundance, and love. Their vibrant color and distinctive shape make them popular motifs in various artistic expressions.

Medicinal and Culinary Uses:

Beyond their symbolic significance, pomegranates were historically valued for their medicinal properties. Ancient civilizations used different parts of the tree, from the bark to the fruit, for remedies to treat various ailments. Today, they are recognized for their nutritional value, packed with antioxidants and vitamins, making them a sought-after fruit for both health and culinary purposes.

Global Influence:

The popularity of pomegranates has transcended borders and time, becoming an integral part of cuisines, customs, and traditions in different parts of the world. From Middle Eastern dishes like tabbouleh and Persian fesenjan to Indian chutneys and Mediterranean salads, the fruit's seeds or juice are incorporated into diverse recipes, showcasing its culinary versatility.

Contemporary Significance:

In modern times, pomegranates continue to hold significance, with increased scientific interest in their health benefits. Their cultivation, aided by advancements in agricultural techniques, has expanded to different climates globally, contributing to their availability year-round and their position as a symbol of health and vitality.

The pomegranate's enduring presence in history, mythology, art, and its continued use in culinary and medicinal practices, solidify its place as a fruit deeply intertwined with human culture, traditions, and symbolism across diverse societies.

1.3 Varieties of Pomegranate Trees

Pomegranates come in various cultivars, each with its unique characteristics in terms of fruit size, taste, color, and adaptability to different climates. Here's an overview of some popular varieties of pomegranate trees:

1. Wonderful:

- **Description:** One of the most well-known commercial cultivars, known for its large, deep red fruits.

- **Attributes:** Sweet and tangy arils with a rich flavor. This variety is often used for juicing due to its high juice content.

- **Growth:** Adaptable to different climates, but it thrives in warmer regions.

2. Haku Botan:

- **Description:** Originating from Japan, it's a dwarf variety with small to medium-sized fruits.

- **Attributes:** Known for its sweet and flavorful arils with a hint of acidity.

- **Growth:** Suitable for smaller spaces or containers, making it popular for home gardens.

3. Eversweet:

- **Description:** A relatively new cultivar, prized for its sweet taste and low acidity.

- **Attributes:** The arils are very sweet and less tart compared to other varieties.

- **Growth:** Tolerant of cooler climates, making it a suitable choice for regions with milder winters.

4. Parfianka:

- **Description:** Originating from Turkmenistan, this cultivar produces medium to large fruits.

- **Attributes:** Known for its complex, rich flavor profile with a good balance of sweetness and acidity.

- **Growth:** Requires a longer growing season, making it more suitable for warmer climates.

5. Nana:

- **Description:** A dwarf variety, ideal for small gardens or containers.

- **Attributes:** Produces small to medium-sized fruits with tangy, flavorful arils.

- **Growth:** Well-suited for cooler climates and can thrive in containers, making it adaptable to various environments.

6. Ambrosia:

- **Description:** A newer variety known for its exceptionally sweet and juicy arils.

- **Attributes:** Very sweet with minimal tartness, making it popular for fresh consumption.

- **Growth:** Thrives in warm climates and requires sufficient sunlight for optimal fruit development.

7. Cloud:

- **Description:** This variety is recognized for its pale pink to white arils.

- **Attributes:** Delicate, sweet taste with subtle acidity, prized for its unique color.

- **Growth:** Suited for warm climates and needs proper care to achieve optimal fruit coloration.

8. Angel Red:

- **Description:** A dwarf variety producing small to medium-sized deep red fruits.

- **Attributes:** Sweet and tangy arils with a balanced flavor profile.

- **Growth:** Ideal for smaller gardens or containers, adaptable to various climates.

These varieties showcase the diversity within the pomegranate species, offering a range of flavors, sizes, and adaptability to different environmental conditions. Choosing the right variety depends on factors like climate, space availability, taste preferences, and intended use (fresh consumption or juicing).

1.3 Benefits of Pomegranate Trees

The pomegranate tree is also valued for its versatility. Its fruits can be consumed fresh, juiced, or used in cooking, lending their sweet-tart flavor to various dishes, from salads to desserts, and even savory recipes. Pomegranate juice, rich in antioxidants, is a popular beverage choice, revered for its health-boosting properties.

Beyond its culinary significance, the pomegranate tree holds cultural and symbolic importance in many societies. In some cultures, the fruit is a symbol of fertility, prosperity, and good fortune. Its prominence in ancient mythology and religious texts, often representing life, regeneration, and abundance, underscores its cultural significance across civilizations.

The pomegranate tree isn't solely valuable for its fruit; it plays a vital role in the ecosystem. Its vibrant flowers attract pollinators like bees, contributing to biodiversity and the health of surrounding flora. Additionally, the tree's resilience in various climates and its ability to thrive in arid regions make it a valuable asset in sustainable agriculture and reforestation efforts.

The pomegranate tree is lauded for its medicinal properties. Various parts of the tree, including the bark, roots, and leaves, have been utilized in traditional medicine for their potential therapeutic effects. They have been historically employed to treat conditions like diarrhea, ulcers, and even certain infections. Additionally, pomegranate extracts and oils are utilized in skincare products for their antioxidant and anti-inflammatory properties, promoting healthier skin.

Cultivating pomegranate trees also presents economic benefits. They offer opportunities for agricultural livelihoods, with the fruit's demand in the global market continually increasing due to its health-conscious consumer base.

Health-wise, the pomegranate's contributions are continually being researched and unveiled. Studies suggest that compounds found in pomegranates might aid in combating inflammation, oxidative stress, and even neurological conditions. Some research indicates potential benefits for brain health, including protection against Alzheimer's disease and improved memory function due to the fruit's neuroprotective properties.

pomegranate-derived supplements or extracts have shown promise in promoting cardiovascular health. They may help lower cholesterol levels, reduce arterial plaque buildup, and enhance overall heart function, contributing to a decreased risk of heart disease and stroke.

The fruit's role in digestive health shouldn't be overlooked either. Pomegranates contain dietary fiber, which aids in digestion and may alleviate symptoms of gastrointestinal disorders. The high fiber content can help regulate bowel movements and promote a healthy gut microbiome, supporting overall digestive well-being.

From a scientific perspective, the pomegranate tree holds fascination. Researchers are exploring its genetic makeup to enhance cultivation practices, improve fruit yield, and develop disease-resistant varieties. Understanding the tree's genetics can also aid in preserving biodiversity and developing more sustainable agricultural methods.

The tree's resilience in adverse conditions makes it an attractive option for agroforestry and reforestation initiatives. Its ability to withstand drought conditions and poor soil quality allows it to thrive in regions where other crops might struggle, thereby aiding in soil conservation and ecosystem restoration.

In the realm of industry, pomegranate byproducts find diverse applications.

Pomegranate peel, often considered waste, contains bioactive compounds that can be utilized in producing dyes, natural pesticides, and animal feed supplements, reducing environmental waste and promoting a circular economy.

The oil extracted from pomegranate seeds is rich in fatty acids and antioxidants, making it a valuable ingredient in cosmetic and skincare products. It's utilized in moisturizers, serums, and lotions for its anti-aging and skin-rejuvenating properties, contributing to the thriving cosmetics industry.

The pomegranate tree's benefits ripple across various fields, from health and science to environmental conservation and industry. Its remarkable qualities continue to unveil new possibilities, making it an invaluable asset to both human well-being and the planet's ecosystem.

CHAPTER 2

Growing Conditions

2.1 Climate Requirements

Pomegranate trees thrive in a variety of climates, but they have specific preferences when it comes to temperature, sunlight, and humidity. Understanding their climate requirements is crucial for successful cultivation:

Temperature:

- **Warm Summers:** Pomegranates prefer warm to hot summers for optimal fruit production. They thrive in regions where temperatures consistently reach between

77°F to 90°F (25°C to 32°C) during the growing season.

- **Chilling Hours:** Some varieties require a period of winter chill (between 100 to 200 hours below 45°F or 7°C) to stimulate flowering and fruiting. However, certain cultivars are more adaptable to milder winters.

Frost and Cold Tolerance:

- **Cold Hardy Varieties:** Certain cultivars, like 'Wonderful' and 'Parfianka,' exhibit good cold tolerance and can withstand temperatures down to 10°F (-12°C) once established.

- **Protection from Frost:** Young trees are more susceptible to frost damage, so in areas with occasional frost, providing

protection during winter is
advisable.

Sunlight:

- **Full Sunlight:** Pomegranate
  trees thrive in full sun,
  requiring at least 6 to 8 hours of
  direct sunlight daily for optimal
  growth, fruiting, and
  sweetening of the fruit.

- **Sheltered Locations:** While
  they enjoy sunlight, young trees
  benefit from some protection
  against strong winds or extreme
  heat, especially in arid regions.

Soil and Humidity:

- **Well-Drained Soil:**
  Pomegranates prefer well-
  draining soil to avoid
  waterlogging, which can cause
  root rot. Sandy loam or loamy

soils with good drainage are ideal.

- **Moderate Humidity:** They tolerate a range of humidity levels but prefer drier conditions during the fruiting season to minimize issues with fruit cracking and diseases.

Climate Adaptability:

- **Adaptable Trees:** Certain cultivars have varying degrees of adaptability to different climates. Some are more suitable for tropical or subtropical regions, while others thrive in more temperate climates with distinct seasons.

Understanding the specific climate needs of pomegranate trees allows growers to select appropriate cultivars and provide the necessary care and environmental conditions for healthy growth, flowering, and fruit production. Adjustments in cultivation techniques can also help mitigate challenges posed by climate variations in different regions.

2.2 Soil Preparation and pH Levels

Preparing the soil and maintaining appropriate pH levels are crucial steps in successfully cultivating pomegranate trees. Here's a guide to soil preparation and pH requirements:

Soil Preparation:

1. **Well-Drained Soil:** Pomegranates thrive in well-drained soil to prevent waterlogging. Sandy loam or loamy soils with good drainage

are ideal. Amending heavy clay soils with organic matter can improve drainage.

2. **pH Levels:** Aim for a slightly acidic to neutral pH range between 5.5 to 7.0. Conduct a soil test to determine the pH of your soil before planting.

3. **Soil Enrichment:** Prior to planting, enrich the soil with compost, aged manure, or organic matter. This helps improve soil structure, fertility, and moisture retention.

4. **Weed Control:** Remove weeds and debris from the planting area to reduce competition for nutrients and water.

pH Levels:

1. **Testing Soil pH:** Use a soil pH testing kit or send a sample to a local agricultural extension service for analysis. This helps determine the soil's acidity or alkalinity.

2. **Acidic Soil Adjustments:** If the soil pH is too high (alkaline), amendments like elemental sulfur or acidifying fertilizers can lower the pH gradually. Incorporating peat moss or pine needles also helps increase acidity.

3. **Alkaline Soil Adjustments:** To raise pH levels in overly acidic soil, adding agricultural lime or dolomitic lime can help balance the acidity over time.

Planting Considerations:

1. **Planting Depth:** When
   planting pomegranate trees,
   ensure they are placed at the
   same depth as they were in
   their nursery containers.
   Planting too deep can cause
   issues with root rot.

2. **Spacing:** Provide adequate
   space between trees to allow for
   proper growth and airflow.
   Space standard varieties around
   12 to 15 feet apart and dwarf
   varieties around 6 to 10 feet
   apart.

3. **Mulching:** Mulch around the
   base of the tree with organic
   mulch like wood chips or straw
   to retain moisture, suppress
   weeds, and regulate soil
   temperature.

Maintenance:

Regularly monitor the soil's moisture levels, especially during the tree's establishment phase. Water deeply but infrequently to encourage deeper root growth. Periodic soil testing helps ensure the pH remains within the optimal range for healthy pomegranate tree growth.

focusing on soil preparation, adjusting pH levels as needed, and providing proper planting conditions, you set the groundwork for healthy root development and overall tree vigor, leading to better fruit production and tree resilience.

2.3 Sunlight and Watering Needs

Understanding the sunlight requirements and proper watering practices is essential for nurturing healthy and productive pomegranate trees:

Sunlight Needs:

1. **Full Sun Exposure:** Pomegranate trees thrive in full sunlight, requiring at least 6 to 8 hours of direct sunlight per day for optimal growth and fruit production.

2. **Sunlight for Fruit Development:** Adequate sunlight exposure is crucial during the fruiting season as it helps the fruit develop its characteristic color, sweetness, and overall flavor.

3. **Protection from Extreme Heat:** While they love sunlight, young trees might benefit from some protection during intense heatwaves, especially in arid

regions. Providing shade or temporary shields can prevent stress on young plants.

Watering Needs:

1. **Establishment Phase:** During the first year or two after planting, young pomegranate trees require regular watering to establish deep root systems. Water deeply but infrequently, ensuring the soil remains consistently moist but not waterlogged.

2. **Mature Trees:** Once established, pomegranate trees are relatively drought-tolerant. However, they still benefit from periodic deep watering, especially during hot and dry spells.

3. **Seasonal Watering:** Adjust watering frequency based on the season. Increase watering during the flowering and fruiting seasons to support healthy fruit development. Reduce watering in the dormant winter period to prevent root rot in cold, wet soils.

4. **Soil Moisture Check:** Use a moisture meter or check soil moisture levels by digging a few inches deep around the tree. Water when the top few inches of soil feel dry.

Watering Tips:

1. **Deep Watering:** Encourage deep root growth by applying water slowly and deeply, allowing it to penetrate the root

zone rather than surface watering.

2. **Mulching:** Mulch around the base of the tree helps retain soil moisture, reduces evaporation, and regulates soil temperature. This assists in maintaining consistent moisture levels.

3. **Avoid Waterlogging:** Ensure proper drainage to prevent waterlogging, as excessive moisture can lead to root rot and other issues.

4. **Rainfall Consideration:** Adjust watering schedules based on natural rainfall. During rainy periods, reduce supplemental watering to prevent oversaturation.

Observing the Tree:

Regularly observe the tree for signs of stress such as wilting, drooping leaves, or leaf curling, which might indicate insufficient or excess watering. Adjust watering practices accordingly to meet the tree's needs based on environmental conditions and growth stages.

providing adequate sunlight exposure and practicing proper watering techniques tailored to the tree's age and environmental conditions, you support healthy growth, robust fruit development, and overall tree vigor.

CHAPTER 3

Planting and Care

3.1 Planting Pomegranate Trees

Planting pomegranate trees involves several key steps to ensure proper establishment and healthy growth. Here's a comprehensive guide:

Timing:

1. **Season:** The best time to plant pomegranate trees is in late winter to early spring, preferably after the last frost date in your region. This allows the tree to establish roots before the growing season begins.

Steps for Planting:

1. **Selecting a Location:**

    - Choose a site with full sunlight exposure (6 to 8 hours of direct sunlight daily).

    - Ensure well-drained soil, preferably sandy loam or loamy soil with good drainage.

2. **Preparing the Planting Hole:**

    - Dig a hole that is twice as wide but just as deep as the root ball or nursery container.

    - Loosen the soil in the hole and mix in organic matter like compost or aged manure.

3. **Removing the Tree from the Container:**

- Gently remove the tree from its container by tapping or squeezing the sides of the container. Avoid pulling on the tree.

4. **Placing the Tree in the Hole:**

   - Set the tree in the center of the hole at the same depth it was planted in the container.

   - Ensure the tree is upright and its root flare (where the roots meet the trunk) is at ground level.

5. **Backfilling and Watering:**

   - Fill the hole with soil, firmly packing it around the roots while avoiding air pockets.

- Water thoroughly to settle the soil and eliminate air pockets.

6. **Mulching and Support:**

   - Apply a layer of organic mulch around the base of the tree, keeping it a few inches away from the trunk.

   - Use stakes or ties if the tree requires support against strong winds or if it's a bare-root tree.

7. **Watering and Care:**

   - Water the newly planted tree deeply immediately after planting and continue to water regularly, especially during the establishment phase.

- Prune back any broken or damaged branches and maintain a balanced shape.

Spacing and Considerations:

- **Spacing:** Space standard pomegranate trees around 12 to 15 feet apart and dwarf varieties around 6 to 10 feet apart to allow for proper growth and airflow.

- **Pollination:** Some varieties may require cross-pollination for better fruit set, so consider planting multiple compatible varieties if necessary.

- **Protection:** Provide temporary shade or cover during extreme heat or cold for young trees to prevent stress.

After Planting Care:

- **Monitoring:** Regularly check soil moisture and adjust watering as needed, ensuring the soil remains consistently moist but not waterlogged.

- **Fertilization:** Avoid fertilizing newly planted trees immediately; wait until the tree shows signs of new growth before applying a balanced fertilizer.

By following these steps and providing proper care, you set the stage for a strong foundation that promotes healthy root development and vigorous growth in your pomegranate tree.

3.2 Pruning Techniques

Pruning plays a crucial role in shaping the growth, promoting fruit production, and maintaining the health of pomegranate trees. Here are some pruning techniques and tips:

Timing of Pruning:

1. **Winter Pruning:** The best time for major pruning is during late winter or early spring, while the tree is still dormant before new growth begins. This timing allows the tree to recover and encourages vigorous growth in the upcoming season.

Techniques for Pruning:

1. **Removing Dead or Damaged Branches:**

   - Begin by identifying and removing any dead,

diseased, or damaged
branches. Use clean,
sharp pruning shears or
loppers to make clean
cuts.

2. **Thinning the Canopy:**

    - Thin out crowded or
      crossing branches to
      improve airflow and
      sunlight penetration into
      the center of the tree.
      This reduces the risk of
      disease and encourages
      fruit development.

3. **Shaping and Training:**

    - Shape the tree to a
      desired form, such as an
      open vase or modified
      central leader structure.
      Encourage outward
      growth by cutting back

inward-growing
branches.

4. **Suckers and Water Sprouts:**

- Remove suckers (shoots emerging from the base of the tree) and water sprouts (vertical, fast-growing shoots) regularly to maintain a tidy and productive tree.

5. **Heading Cuts for Height Control:**

- Conduct heading cuts (removing a portion of a branch) to manage the height of the tree if needed. However, avoid excessive pruning of the main branches, as it can affect fruit production.

6. **Selective Pruning for Fruit
    Production:**

    - Prune to encourage fruit-
      bearing wood by
      favoring strong, healthy
      branches that are capable
      of bearing fruit. Remove
      excess growth that
      doesn't contribute to
      fruiting.

Tips for Pruning:

- **Tools:** Use sharp and clean
  pruning tools to make smooth
  cuts that heal faster and reduce
  the risk of disease transmission.

- **Moderation:** Avoid over-
  pruning, as excessive removal
  of branches can stress the tree
  and reduce fruiting potential.

- **Sanitization:** Disinfect pruning tools between cuts, especially when dealing with diseased branches, to prevent the spread of infections.

Post-Pruning Care:

- **Aftercare:** After pruning, monitor the tree for any signs of stress or disease. Ensure proper irrigation and nutrition to support recovery and new growth.

Pruning practices may vary based on the tree's age, variety, growth habit, and regional climate. It's beneficial to familiarize yourself with specific pruning techniques suitable for the type of pomegranate tree you have and adjust your approach accordingly. Regular, thoughtful pruning helps maintain the health, shape, and productivity of your pomegranate tree over time.

3.3 Pest and Disease Management

Managing pests and diseases is crucial for maintaining the health and productivity of pomegranate trees. Here are strategies for pest and disease management:

Common Pests:

1. **Aphids and Whiteflies:**

   - Control aphids and whiteflies by spraying with insecticidal soap or neem oil. Introduce natural predators like ladybugs to help manage aphid populations.

2. **Pomegranate Butterfly (Virachola Isocrates):**

   - Monitor for caterpillars and handpick them if feasible. Use biological control methods or targeted insecticides if infestations are severe.

3. **Fruit Borer (Eudocima Fullonia):**

   - Inspect fruits regularly for signs of larvae entry. Prune and remove affected fruits, and apply insecticides during the egg-laying period.

4. **Scale Insects:**

   - Apply horticultural oil or insecticidal soap to control scale infestations.

Prune and destroy
heavily infested
branches.

Common Diseases:

1. **Fungal Diseases (such as
   Anthracnose and Botrytis):**

   - Promote good airflow by
     proper pruning to reduce
     humidity and prevent
     fungal infections. Apply
     copper-based fungicides
     during the dormant
     season as a preventive
     measure.

2. **Bacterial Blight:**

   - Prune and destroy
     infected branches. Apply
     copper-based sprays
     during the dormant

season to manage bacterial blight.

3. Root Rot (Phytophthora):

- Ensure well-draining soil to prevent waterlogging and root rot. Avoid overwatering and improve soil drainage if necessary.

4. Leaf Spot Diseases:

- Practice good sanitation by removing fallen leaves and debris to reduce disease spread. Apply fungicides as preventive measures during favorable conditions.

Preventive Measures:

1. **Sanitation:** Keep the area
   around the tree clean by
   removing fallen leaves, fruit,
   and debris to minimize disease
   spread.

2. **Healthy Soil and Nutrition:**
   Maintain proper soil pH,
   fertility, and drainage to
   promote tree vigor and
   resilience against diseases.

3. **Pruning Practices:** Prune to
   improve airflow within the
   canopy, reducing humidity and
   limiting conditions favorable
   for disease development.

4. **Monitoring:** Regularly inspect
   the tree for signs of pests or
   diseases, such as wilting,
   discoloration, spots, or
   abnormal growth, to address
   issues promptly.

Integrated Pest Management (IPM):

- **IPM Approach:** Implement an integrated pest management strategy that combines cultural practices, biological controls, and targeted use of pesticides only when necessary, minimizing environmental impact.

- **Natural Predators:** Encourage natural predators like ladybugs, lacewings, or predatory mites to control pest populations as part of an eco-friendly approach.

employing a combination of preventive measures, regular monitoring, and targeted treatments, you can effectively manage pests and diseases, safeguarding the health and

productivity of your pomegranate
trees while minimizing the need for
harsh chemicals.

CHAPTER 4

Pomegranate Tree Maintenance

4.1 Fertilization and Mulching

Maintaining proper fertilization and mulching practices is essential for the health, growth, and fruit production of pomegranate trees.

Fertilization:

1. **Timing:** Apply fertilizer in early spring before new growth begins and again in late spring or early summer after flowering.

2. **Fertilizer Type:** Use a balanced fertilizer or a

formulation specifically designed for fruit trees. Look for options with a ratio close to 10-10-10 or 8-8-8, ensuring a mix of nitrogen (N), phosphorus (P), and potassium (K) along with micronutrients.

3. **Amount:** Follow the manufacturer's instructions for the appropriate amount based on the tree's age and size. Typically, young trees require less fertilizer compared to mature ones.

4. **Application:** Spread the fertilizer evenly around the tree's drip line (the area directly below the outer edges of the canopy) and water thoroughly afterward to allow the nutrients to reach the root zone.

5. **Organic Options:** Consider using organic fertilizers like compost, aged manure, or organic blends to provide slow-release nutrients and improve soil health over time.

Mulching:

1. **Benefits:** Mulching helps conserve soil moisture, suppress weeds, regulate soil temperature, and improve soil structure.

2. **Mulch Type:** Use organic mulch materials such as wood chips, straw, shredded bark, or compost. Apply a layer about 2 to 4 inches thick around the base of the tree, leaving space around the trunk to prevent moisture-related issues.

3. **Application:** Spread mulch evenly around the tree, extending it to the dripline but keeping it away from direct contact with the trunk.

4. **Renewal:** Periodically replenish mulch as it decomposes to maintain the desired thickness. Avoid piling mulch against the trunk, which can promote rot.

5. **Seasonal Considerations:** Adjust the mulch layer thickness to protect the roots from extreme temperatures in summer and winter.

Considerations:

- **Soil Moisture:** Mulching helps retain soil moisture, reducing the frequency of watering. However, ensure proper drainage to prevent waterlogging.

- **Weed Control:** Mulch suppresses weed growth, reducing competition for nutrients and water around the tree's root zone.

- **Avoid Over-Mulching:** While mulch is beneficial, excessive mulching can create an environment prone to pests and diseases. Maintain an appropriate thickness and distance from the trunk.

Regularly fertilizing and mulching your pomegranate tree helps provide essential nutrients, conserves moisture, and maintains a healthy soil environment, promoting optimal growth, flowering, and fruit production. Adjustments in fertilization amounts or mulching frequency may be needed based on soil conditions and the tree's overall health.

4.2 Watering Schedule

Creating a proper watering schedule is crucial for maintaining the health and productivity of pomegranate trees, ensuring they receive adequate moisture without being waterlogged. Here's a guide to a watering schedule:

Watering Guidelines:

1. **Establishment Phase:**

   - Young trees (first 1-2 years): Water deeply and regularly to establish a strong root system. Provide enough moisture to keep the soil

consistently moist but
not waterlogged.

2. **Mature Trees:**

    - Once established,
      pomegranate trees are
      relatively drought-
      tolerant. However, they
      still need regular
      watering, especially
      during dry periods and
      hot seasons.

Watering Techniques:

1. **Deep Watering:** Encourage
    deep root growth by watering
    thoroughly. Apply water slowly
    to allow it to penetrate the soil
    deeply rather than surface
    watering.

2. **Frequency:** Water mature trees
    deeply but infrequently.

Generally, a deep watering session once every 1-2 weeks during dry periods should suffice, but adjust based on soil conditions and weather.

3. **Moisture Check:** Use a moisture meter or check soil moisture by digging a few inches deep around the tree. Water when the top few inches of soil feel dry.

4. **Root Zone Coverage:** Ensure the entire root zone, extending beyond the drip line, receives water. This encourages root expansion and efficient water uptake.

Seasonal Adjustments:

1. **Spring and Summer:**

- Increase watering during active growth, flowering, and fruit development. Supplement with more water during hot and dry spells.

2. **Fall and Winter:**

   - Reduce watering as the tree enters dormancy. Allow the soil to dry slightly between watering sessions, especially in cooler regions.

Factors Affecting Watering:

1. **Soil Type:** Adjust watering frequency based on soil type. Well-draining soils may require more frequent watering compared to heavier clay soils.

2. **Climate:** Consider regional climate conditions, including rainfall patterns and temperature fluctuations, when determining the watering schedule.

3. **Tree Health:** Monitor the tree for signs of stress, such as wilting or leaf drop, which may indicate inadequate watering.

4. **Mulching:** Mulch around the tree helps retain soil moisture, reducing the frequency of watering required.

Note:

- **Balanced Approach:** Avoid both overwatering and underwatering. Overwatering can lead to root rot and other issues, while underwatering can stress the tree and reduce fruit production.

- **Adaptability:** Adjust the watering schedule based on the tree's age, soil conditions, climate, and specific needs. Observing the tree's response to watering helps fine-tune the schedule for optimal growth and health.

4.3 Seasonal Care Tips

Seasonal care for pomegranate trees involves adjusting practices and addressing specific needs during different seasons to support healthy growth and fruit production. Here are seasonal care tips:

Spring:

1. **Fertilization:** Apply a balanced fertilizer early in spring before new growth begins to provide essential nutrients for the upcoming growing season.

2. **Pruning:** Conduct major pruning during late winter or early spring while the tree is still dormant. Remove dead or diseased branches and shape the tree as needed.

3. **Watering:** Ensure adequate soil moisture as the tree enters the growing season, especially if rainfall is scarce.

4. **Pest and Disease Monitoring:** Regularly inspect the tree for signs of pests, diseases, or early leafing. Address issues promptly to prevent spread.

Summer:

1. **Watering:** Increase watering frequency during hot and dry periods to support fruit development. Deep watering helps maintain soil moisture levels.

2. **Mulching:** Maintain a mulch layer to conserve soil moisture, regulate temperature, and suppress weed growth.

3. **Thinning Fruit:** If needed, thin out excessive fruit to promote larger and healthier fruits. Remove small or damaged fruits to allocate resources to the remaining ones.

4. **Protection from Heat:** Provide shade or temporary shields to young trees during extreme heatwaves to prevent sunburn and stress.

Fall:

1. **Watering:** Reduce watering gradually as temperatures cool and the tree prepares for dormancy. Allow the soil to dry slightly between watering sessions.

2. **Harvesting:** Depending on the variety, pomegranates may ripen in fall. Harvest ripe fruits carefully to avoid damage.

3. **Pruning:** Conduct minor pruning as needed, removing any unwanted growth or dead branches. Avoid major pruning, as this may affect next season's growth.

4. **Soil Amendments:** Apply organic matter or compost around the base of the tree to enrich the soil before winter.

Winter:

1. **Protection from Cold:** Provide protection for young trees or those in colder regions against frost or freezing temperatures, especially during the first few winters.

2. **Monitoring:** Monitor the tree for signs of winter damage, such as frostbite or root exposure. Address any issues promptly.

3. **Dormancy Period:** Pomegranate trees enter dormancy during winter. Reduce watering but ensure the tree does not become overly dry.

4. **Planning and Preparation:** Use the dormant season for planning and preparing for the

upcoming growing season, including ordering supplies or considering any necessary changes in care practices.

Note:

- **Adaptation:** Adjust care practices based on regional climate variations and the specific needs of your pomegranate tree. Regular monitoring and attentive care throughout the seasons promote tree health and fruitfulness.

CHAPTER 5

Harvesting and Uses

5.1 Recognizing When Pomegranates are Ready

Recognizing the right time to harvest pomegranates is essential for ensuring the fruit reaches its peak flavor, sweetness, and ripeness. Here are signs to look for when determining if pomegranates are ready for harvest:

External Indicators:

1. **Color Change:** Pomegranates typically change color as they ripen. Look for a vibrant and consistent color—varieties may show a shift from green to shades of red, pink, or yellow depending on the cultivar.

2. **Texture:** The fruit's outer skin should feel firm and have a smooth texture. Ripe pomegranates might have a slightly glossy appearance.

3. **Size and Shape:** Most pomegranate varieties maintain a consistent size and shape when ripe. Check for uniformity and avoid fruits with irregular shapes or sizes.

4. **Cracking:** Be cautious of overripe fruits; excessive ripeness can cause cracking or splitting of the skin, indicating it might be past its prime for optimal taste.

Internal Indicators:

1. **Sound:** A ripe pomegranate often produces a metallic or bell-like sound when tapped

gently, suggesting the arils inside are plump and juicy.

2. **Weight:** The fruit should feel heavy for its size, indicating the abundance of juice-filled arils within.

3. **Aril Color:** Some varieties display a deeper, more intense color of the arils inside when fully ripe. A deep red to burgundy hue is often a good indicator of ripeness.

Time Considerations:

- Depending on the variety, pomegranates usually ripen from late summer to early winter, with harvesting typically occurring from September to December in many regions.

Note:

- Pomegranates do not ripen further once harvested. It's essential to pick them at the right time to ensure optimal flavor and quality.

Observing these indicators collectively helps determine the right time for harvesting pomegranates, ensuring the best taste and quality for consumption or processing.

5.2 Harvesting Techniques

Harvesting pomegranates requires care to avoid damaging the fruit and to ensure they're picked at the right time for the best flavor and quality. Here are techniques for harvesting pomegranates:

Timing:

- **Ripe Stage:** Harvest pomegranates when they reach their peak color and size, displaying external indicators like color change and a firm texture.

Harvesting Techniques:

1. **Cutting Technique:**

   - Use sharp pruning shears or scissors to cut the fruit from the tree. Leave a small portion of the stem attached to the fruit.

2. **Twist and Pull Method:**

   - Gently twist and pull the pomegranate from the tree, ensuring it detaches easily without damaging the stem or the fruit.

3. **Avoid Pulling:**

- Avoid pulling forcefully or yanking the fruit, as it may damage the stem or cause the fruit to split.

4. **Handling Care:**

   - Handle the harvested fruits carefully to prevent bruising or damage to the skin, which can affect storage life and quality.

Precautions and Tips:

1. **Gentle Handling:** Handle the fruit delicately to prevent bruising or puncturing, as damaged pomegranates are prone to spoilage.

2. **Inspecting Each Fruit:** Inspect each harvested fruit to ensure it's ripe and free from damage or signs of rotting.

3. **Stem Preservation:** Leaving a small part of the stem attached to the fruit helps prolong its shelf life.

4. **Basket or Container:** Use shallow baskets or containers lined with soft padding or cloth to prevent the fruits from rubbing against each other.

5. **Harvest Timing:** Aim to harvest in the morning when temperatures are cooler, which helps maintain the fruit's freshness.

Post-Harvest Handling:

- After harvesting, store the pomegranates in a cool, dry place or refrigerate them if not using immediately. Proper storage prolongs their shelf life.

Note:

- Pomegranates don't ripen further once harvested. Ensure you pick them at the right stage of ripeness to enjoy their optimal taste and quality.

Following these harvesting techniques ensures that pomegranates are picked at their peak, preserving their flavor and quality for consumption or processing.

5.3 Culinary and Medicinal Uses

Pomegranates offer a versatile range of culinary and medicinal uses, showcasing their flavorful arils, nutrient-rich juice, and beneficial properties. Here are some ways they're utilized:

Culinary Uses:

1. **Fresh Consumption:**

   - Enjoy the arils fresh as a snack or in salads, adding a burst of sweet-tart flavor and a crunchy texture.

2. **Juicing:**

   - Extract the juice from the arils to create refreshing beverages, smoothies, or cocktails. Pomegranate juice is prized for its vibrant color and health benefits.

3. **Sauces and Dressings:**

   - Use pomegranate juice or arils to create flavorful sauces, marinades, or salad dressings, adding

depth and a tangy
sweetness to dishes.

4. **Desserts:**

- Incorporate arils or juice
  into desserts such as
  cakes, tarts, sorbets, or as
  a topping for yogurt or
  ice cream.

5. **Preserves and Jams:**

- Create preserves, jams,
  or jellies with the juice or
  arils, adding a unique
  twist to spreads or
  glazes.

Medicinal Uses:

1. **Antioxidant Properties:**

- Pomegranates are rich in
  antioxidants, particularly
  polyphenols, which may

help protect against free radicals and promote overall health.

2. **Heart Health:**

   - Studies suggest that pomegranate consumption may support heart health by improving cholesterol levels and reducing blood pressure.

3. **Anti-Inflammatory Effects:**

   - Some research indicates that pomegranates have anti-inflammatory properties that could benefit conditions like arthritis and other inflammatory diseases.

4. **Digestive Health:**

- Pomegranates contain dietary fiber, aiding digestion and potentially reducing the risk of digestive issues.

5. **Potential Anti-Cancer Properties:**

   - Certain studies suggest that compounds in pomegranates may have anticancer effects, though more research is needed in this area.

Traditional and Cultural Uses:

- In various cultures, pomegranates symbolize fertility, abundance, and prosperity. They're often included in rituals, ceremonies, and traditional medicines.

Precautions:

- While pomegranates offer numerous health benefits, individuals on specific medications or with certain health conditions should consult a healthcare professional before significantly increasing their pomegranate intake, as it may interact with medications or exacerbate certain health issues.

From culinary delights to potential health benefits, pomegranates are prized for their versatility and nutritional value, making them a flavorful addition to both cuisine and wellness practices across cultures.

www.ingramcontent.com/pod-product-compliance
Lightning Source LLC
Chambersburg PA
CBHW050837260726
48660CB00006B/2289